SPEECH PHYSIOLOGY:
Brain centers co-responsible for specific, meaningful, articulate, relevant, & time-bound [S.M.A.R.T.] speech

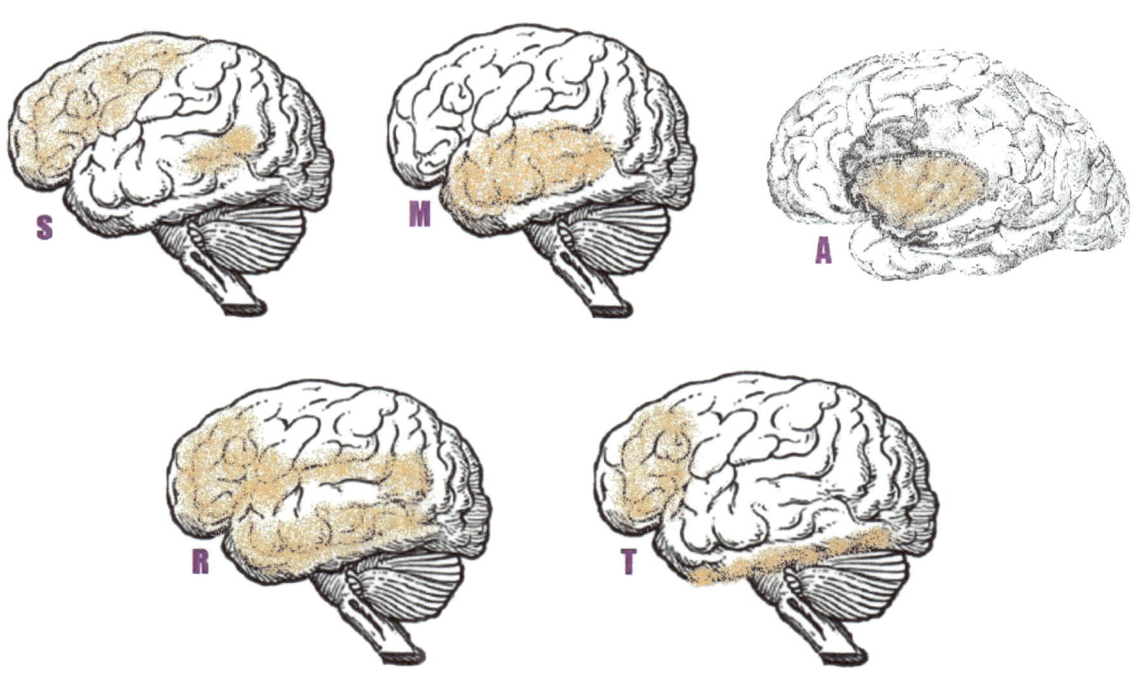

Naira Roland Matevosyan, M.D, Ph.D
Copyright © 2013 with Naira Matevosyan, *"L'auteur" librairie*
ISBN:978-1490358284; CreateSpace, Inc., North Charleston, SC

CONTENTS

Vocabulary spurt	3
Measuring spurt through stochastic simulation	9
Speech centers in brain	19
Prosody	24
Aphasia	29
Polyglotism and Savant syndrome	33
Physiology of the S.M.A.R.T. speech:	41
- Specific speech	42
- Meaningful speech	42
- Articulate speech	43
- Relevant speech	44
- time-bounding speech	47
Conclusions	48
Index of terms	49
Works cited	52

VOCABULARY SPURT

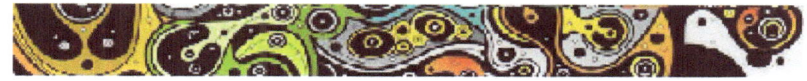

Speech is unique to humans.

The ability to speak is inherent only in the human species with the rare exceptions in some animals (seal, cat, chimpanzee) or birds (parrot) which produce sounds and gestures resembling those of a human language - sometimes with, and sometimes without semantic grounding.

Language is passed from one generation to the next. An infant is born with the ability to learn language but not to speak. Infants' perception of speech is distinct. Between 6 and 10 months of age, infants can discriminate sounds used in the languages of the world. By 10 to 12 months, infants can no longer discriminate between speech sounds that are not used in the language(s) to which they are exposed.

Among 6-month old infants, seen articulations actually enhance their ability to discriminate sounds, and may also contribute to infants' ability to learn phonemic boundaries. Babbling shifts towards meaningful speech as infants grow and produce their first words around the age of one year. In early word learning, infants build their vocabulary slowly.

Children's phonological development normally proceeds as follows:

6–8 weeks: Cooing appears

16 weeks: Laughter and vocal play appear

6–9 months: Reduplicated (canonical) babbling appears

12 months: First words use a limited sound repertoire

18 months: Phonological processes (deformations of target sounds) become systematic.

18 months–7 years: Phonological inventory completion.

Thus, infants' phonological register is completed between the ages of 18 months and 7 years. During that time they add to their vocabulary as they accrue education and experience. There is a relationship between children's prelinguistic phonetic skills and their lexical progress at age two: failure to develop the required phonetic skills in their prelinguistic period results in children's delay in producing words.[1-3]

A switch from an early stage of slow vocabulary growth to a later stage of faster growth is referred to as the *vocabulary spurt*. [4, 5]

A vocabulary spurt often occurs overtime as the number of words learned accelerates. It is believed that most children add about 10 to 20 new words a week. Between the ages of 18 to 24 months, children learn how to combine two words. Three-word and four-word combinations appear when most of the child's utterances are two-word productions. In addition, children are able to form conjoined sentences, using '*and*.' This suggests that there is a vocabulary spurt between the time that the child's first word appears, and when the child is able to form more than two words and eventually, sentences.

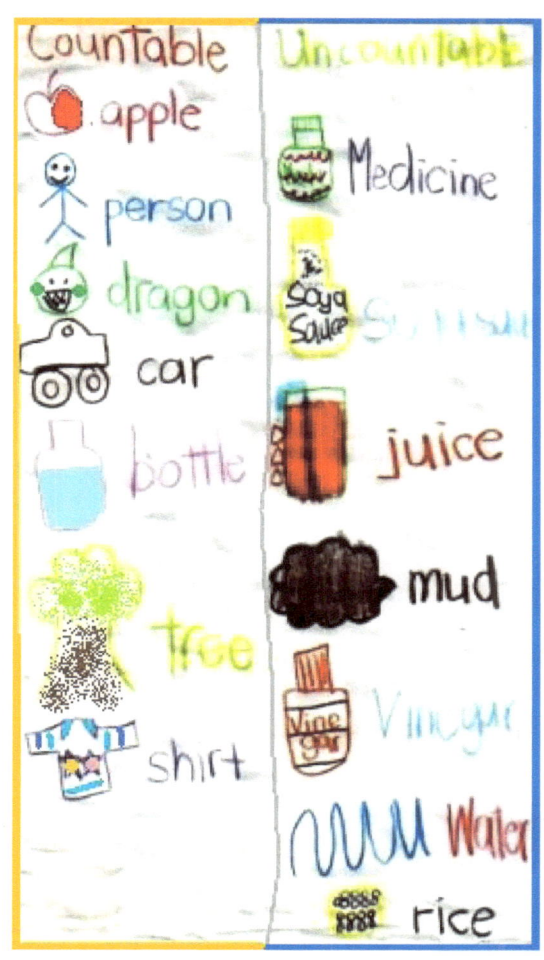

Typically developing children utter their first words between 8 and 14 months of age. At this time, they add words to their repertoire at a slow rate. As they get older and their vocabulary increases, their rate of learning new words also increases—it has to if they are to reach an average vocabulary level of 300 words by 24 months and 60,000 words by 18 years. In addition, it is widely held that children's rate of vocabulary acquisition does not simply increase but undergoes a discrete transition at approximately 50 words. At this time, children putatively switch from an initial stage of slow vocabulary growth to a subsequent stage of faster growth. This transition is seen as the vocabulary spurt, the vocabulary burst, or the naming explosion.

Figure 1: Lexical acquisition norms from the MacArthur-Bates Communicative Development Inventory (MCDI).

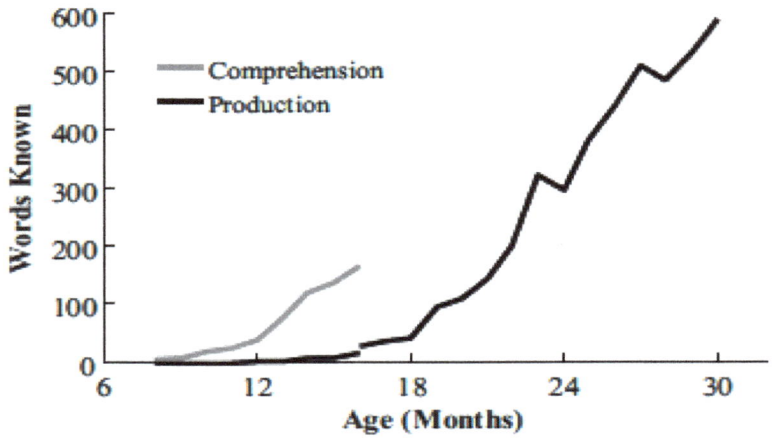

The spurt typically occurs in the second year of life. During this time, the rate of word learning accelerates dramatically (Figure 1). Lexical acquisition norms suggest that between 11 and 15 months of age, children acquire on average 2.7 new words/month, while from 17-21 months, they average 27.9.[6]

By age 5 years, children tend to have an expressive vocabulary of 2,100–2,200 words. By age 6 years, they have approximately 2,600 words of expressive vocabulary and 20,000–24,000 words of receptive vocabulary. From age 6 to 8, the average child in school is learning 6–7 words per day, and from age 8 to 12, approximately 12 words per day.[7,8]

The cause of the spurt was always a subject of much debate. Initial explanations posited a unitary change in the child: the sudden realization that things have names, the onset of categorization abilities, or the acquisition of word learning constraints.[9,10]

Such things would suggest a one-time, stage-like increase in the rate of learning. However, there have been arguments as to whether or not there is a spurt in acquisition of words, for only about one in five children do have a spurt. Using longitudinal data from 38 children, authors modeled the rate of word learning with two functions, one with an inflection point (logistic), which would indicate a spurt, and one without an inflection point (quadratic). Comparing the fits of these two functions using likelihood ratios, they found that just 5 children had a better logistic fit, which indicated that these children underwent a spurt. [4]

While this rules out a one-time developmental event as the cause of the vocabulary explosion, it nevertheless raises the question as to what causes the more general acceleration seen throughout childhood.

A second class of explanations can be termed bootstrapping or leveraged learning approaches. These include mechanisms like segmentation, mutual exclusivity or syntactic bootstrapping. In all three cases, existing words in the lexicon are used to help acquire new words.[11-14]

As each word is learned, these specialized mechanisms become more powerful, enabling faster word learning. Such approaches are supported by computational work. Simple exponential growth systems can model the vocabulary spurt, but only if the rate of change is a function of the number of words already learned.

MEASURING SPURT THROUGH STOCHASTIC SIMULATION

McMurray et al (2007) from Iowa University have demonstrated that acceleration or vocabulary spurt is a mathematical consequence of parallel learning and the statistical distribution of word difficulty across the language. They have generalized this model by developing a stochastic version, which demonstrates that the gradual nature of learning is critical for producing acceleration, and given sufficient gradualness, virtually any distribution of word difficulty can yield acceleration. Thus, the vocabulary explosion may be even more mathematically robust than previously thought.[15]

McMurray and colleagues argue that acceleration is a mathematical by-product of known properties of word learning. It will occur as long as words are learned in parallel and there are fewer easy words than moderately difficult words. This model suggests that specialized word learning mechanisms are not needed to explain acceleration in vocabulary growth (although they may exist to solve other problems).

The generalized stochastic version of the deterministic model taken as a parameter, the authors ask about the relationship between learning history and acceleration. A critical factor in the McMurray model is the distribution of *Gaussian difficulty* across the lexicon. This describes the relative number of easy, moderate and hard words. Given the *G-difficulty* measure, the number of words known at any given time -T, is simply the integral of that distribution from zero to T.

Word-difficulty is likely to be the sum of many factors (phonological complexity, frequency in the child's environment, syntactic category, others). Since these factors will be largely independent, their individual distributions sum to a Gaussian (by the *Central Limit Theorem*). However, any distribution of difficulty which includes only few easy (small *Di*) and more moderate (mid range *Di*) will show acceleration in learning.

A model incorporating some degree of randomness would be more theoretically valid and perhaps more generalizable. The authors[15] introduce a stochastic version of the model which shows not only that the acceleration in word learning is extremely robust but also reveals the importance of learning history. Numbering each word $i = 1$ to N, where N is the number of words to be learned, each word is assigned a difficulty D_i so that the distribution of difficulties approximates G. In the deterministic case, at each time–step one point is added to each word.

When a word reaches its threshold - D_i, it has been learned. To make this model stochastic, the authors again number each word $i = 1$ to N. Each word is assigned a probability - p_i, which is proportional to the frequency of the word. Each word is also assigned a threshold, r_i, the number of repetitions required before a word is learned.

At each time step, a word has probability p_i of gaining a point and it is learned once it has accumulated r_i points. The analysis of the stochastic model is done by first investigating the time to acquisition of a single word, and computation of the cumulative distribution function - $F_i(T)$, for the time of acquisition of that word. So $F_i(T)$ is the probability that the i-word has been learned by time T. Then, the the expected number of words learned are modeled as a function of time - $L(T)$. Since the acquisition of the words is independent, $L(T)$ is the sum of these distributions, F_i. That is:

$$L(T) = \text{expected number of words learned by time } T$$
$$= \sum_i P(\text{the } i^{th} \text{ word was learned by time } T)$$
$$= \sum_i F_i(T)$$

A series of simulations implement the deterministic and stochastic models to compare their performances. Each model is run 10 times using the representative parameters. For each model, a 10,000 word lexicon is initialized. Each word was given a difficulty D_i (time-to-acquisition) randomly chosen from a Gaussian distribution, with a mean of 4000 and standard deviation of 1400. For the stochastic model, these are converted into probabilities ($p_i = 1 / D_i$). Then at each time-step 10,000 random numbers (one for each word) are selected from a uniform distribution ranging from 0 to 1. Any word-i, whose random number is less than its p_i, is deemed learned and removed from further consideration.

Analyses are begun with a single word. For ease of notation, the subscripts on F, D, p and r are temporarily dropped. $E(X) = 1/p$ is equal to D which is equivalent in the two models. While the first moments of time-to-acquisition are equivalent, the second moments are not. In the stochastic model, the variance of the time to acquisition is $Var(X)=$

$(1-p)/p^2$ (it is zero in the deterministic model). Additionally, the coefficient of variation (a non-dimensional measure of the spread of a random variable) is $\sqrt{1-p}$.

Since *p* must necessarily be small (otherwise the model will acquire the bulk of the lexicon within the first measurement period), the variance in time-to-acquisition (*X*) will necessarily be high. Thus, any single run of the model is quite unlikely to approximate the expected values of *X*. In a sense, then, the extreme variance of this model prevents it from modeling difficulty to the same degree as the deterministic model.

The probability that the word is learned at time *T* is simply the probability that that word was not learned on the previous *T* −1 steps times the probability that it is learned on time *T*.

$$p^{(T)} = (1-p)^{T-1}p$$

As such, the probability that a word is learned by time T is:

$$F(T) = \sum_{i=1}^{T} p^{(i)} = 1 - (1-p)^T$$

Intuitively, the rate of change of this function *F* at time *T* is the probability that the word is learned at time *T*. That is $\Delta F/\Delta T = p^{(T)}$. Since $p^{(T)}$ decreases as a function of *T*, *F(T)* is concave down. Thus, the likelihood of learning any given word continually decreases over the life of the model. This explains the failure of this model to show acceleration. The cumulative distribution function for each word is concave down. In order to obtain the function, *L(T)* for the expected number of words learned up to time T, McMurray and et al sum the cumulative distribution functions over all the words in the lexicon:

$$L(T) = \sum_{i=1}^{N} F_i(T).$$

Since the sum of concave down functions is concave down, *L(T)* is concave down, too. This can also be understood by looking at the expected number of new words learned on a particular step. At any time step, the expected number of new words learned is the sum of the probabilities *pi* of the remaining words. As more words are learned, this sum must decrease. Thus the number of new words learned is expected to decrease at each time–step. This is true regardless of how the probabilities *pi* are chosen.

Gradual learning can easily be incorporated into this stochastic model by setting *r* to any value greater than 1. In this case, the value of

r represents the degree of gradualism, or the amount of history that the child must have with a word to acquire it. Once this property is built into the stochastic model, acceleration returns under virtually all circumstances.

In this model, at each step there is a probability p of acquiring a point and the word is learned once r points have been acquired. The number of time steps until the word is learned (X) is a *Negative Binomial Random Variable* with parameters (r,p). The expected time to acquisition is $E(X) = r/p$ and again, we can compare with the deterministic model by setting r and p such that $E(X)$ is the time to acquisition.

To test this, the prior stochastic simulations are repeated, this time with a range of rs (2-20), which is constant for all words within a simulation. Difficulties are selected from an identical Gaussian distribution, and converted to the probability of receiving a point $(p_i = r/D_i)$. This ensures that the mean time-to-acquisition is constant across simulations despite the change in r. Ten simulations are conducted for each r. **Figure 2** shows average vocabulary size as a function of time.

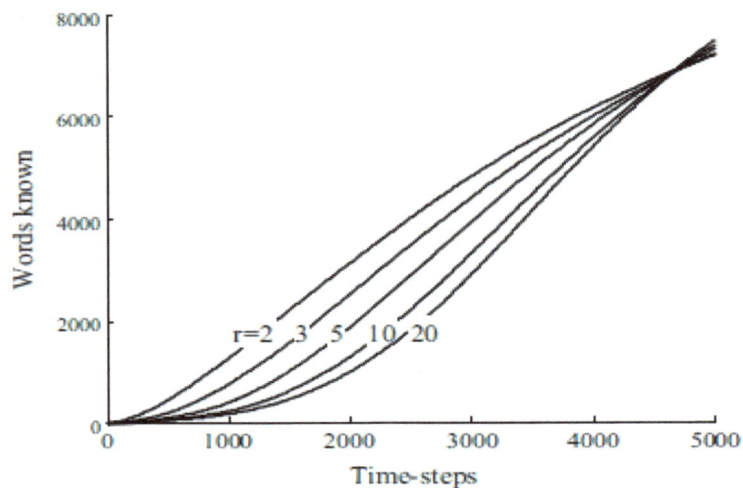

Figure 2: **Vocabulary acquisition in the stochastic model as a function of time and r.**

It is clear that higher values of r show long periods of slow growth followed by acceleration. However, even *r* =2 shows a period of slow growth followed by acceleration. Thus, a vocabulary explosion can be seen as long as *r* > 1.

If *r* > 1, the probability of having learned a word at any given time accelerates. Larger values of *r* increase the suddenness of the acceleration, the length of the acceleration phase (**Figure 3**), and the likelihood that the observed time to acquisition matches the expected. Thus, instantiating history creates a non-deterministic model that captures both parallel learning and difficulty, and hence, shows acceleration.

Figure 3: Results of a stochastic model with a constant p (and by consequence time-to-acquisition, D) across all words.

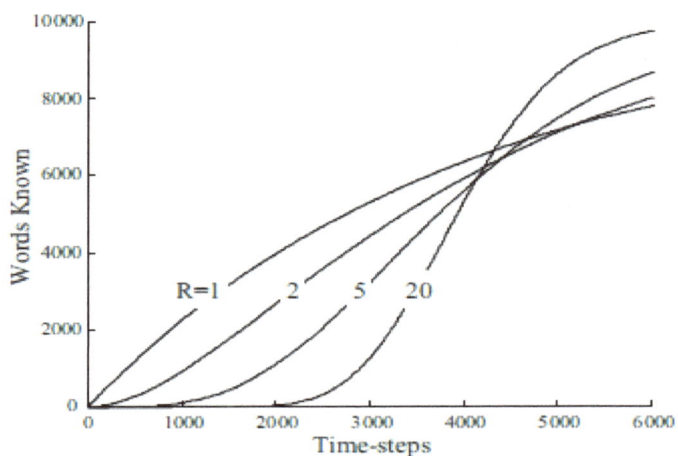

These simulations confirm that the broad framework laid out by McMurray et al, is correct: acceleration in word learning arises out of the mathematical regularities of parallel learning and variation in difficulty. Any stochastic model that incorporates even the minimal amount of gradual learning will show acceleration in word learning.

The only case in which this is not true, is the stochastic model in which learning occurs after a single exposure *(r = 1)*. However, this model does not meaningfully capture learning, and it is not unambiguously parallel.

Overall, the stochastic distribution model suggests that the degree of history required to learn a word is itself a factor in determining the acceleration observed in word learning. Specifically, when learning is very gradual, a substantial spurt can be observed, even when the distribution of easy and hard words does not conform to the assumptions of McMurray.

The vocabulary explosion is an incredibly dramatic developmental process. This has led to a large number of theories positing equally dramatic changes or learning devices on the part of the child. However, such things are not necessary to explain acceleration. Apparent acceleration will always appear in parallel learning systems, even when the fundamental learning processes are perfectly constant. The vocabulary explosion is a mathematically robust phenomenon that will arise under virtually any parallel learning circumstances. There is no need to invoke more complex mechanisms to explain it.

SPEECH CENTERS IN BRAIN

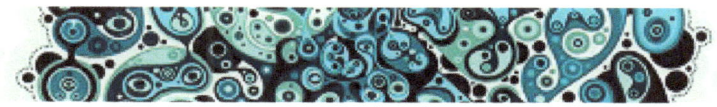

Scientists have long believed that human speech is processed towards the back of the brain's cerebral cortex, behind auditory cortex where all sounds are received: a place known as Wernicke's area. More than 100 imaging studies have updated this information and identified that the speech production center is about 3 centimeters closer to the front of the brain and on the other side of auditory cortex.

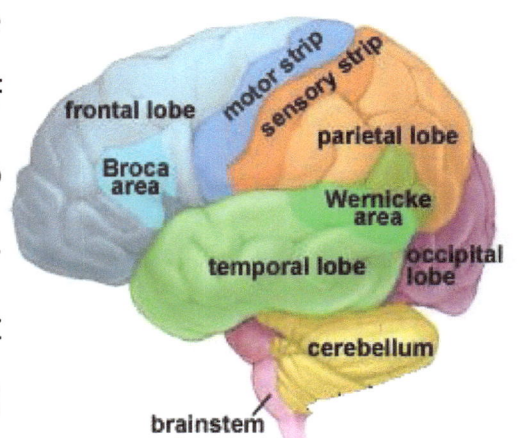

In right-handed individuals the speech center lies in the parietal lobe of the left hemisphere of the brain, also named as the "dominant" hemisphere- responsible for language and speech. It plays a large part in interpreting visual information and spatial processing.

In about one third of individuals who are left-handed, speech function may be located on the right side of the brain. Left-handed individuals may need special testing to determine if their speech center is on the left or right side prior to any surgery in that area.

With the help of blood-oxygen-level-dependent (BOLD) contrasting or magnetic imaging techniques, such Positron Emission Tomography (PET) and Functional Magnetic Resonance Imaging (fMRI), researchers were able to generate pictures showing which areas of a living brain are active at a given time. In the past, research was primarily based on observations of speech functionality in the cerebral cortex. Subcortical regions, such as putamen and the caudate nucleus, as well as the pre-motor areas, among them the Brodmann area-6 (BA6) have received increased attention.[16-18]

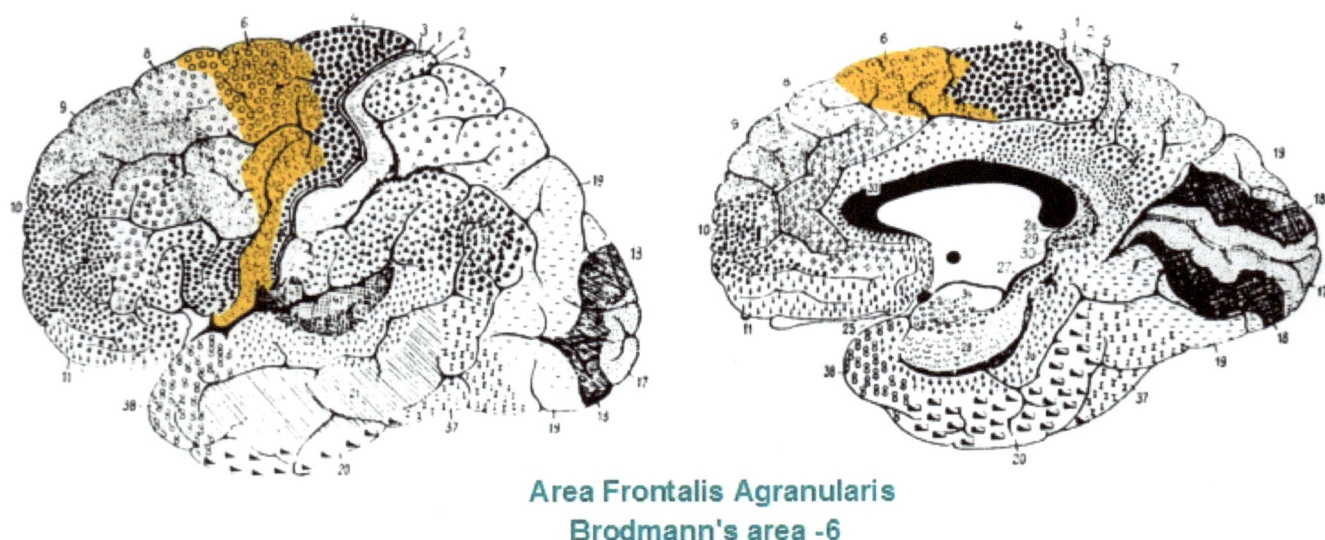

Area Frontalis Agranularis
Brodmann's area -6

It is now generally assumed that the following structures of the cerebral cortex near the primary and secondary auditory cortexes play a fundamental role in speech processing:

- **Superior temporal gyrus (STG)**: morphosyntactic processing (anterior section), integration of syntactic and semantic information (posterior section).

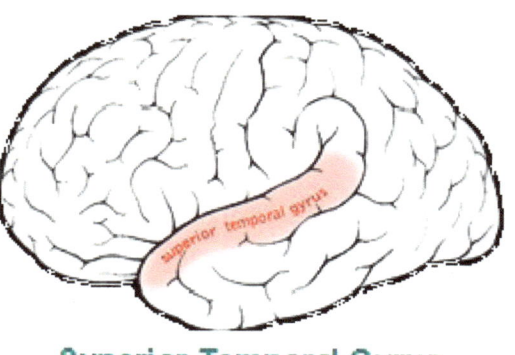
Superior Temporal Gyrus

- **Inferior frontal gyrus (IFG, Brodmann area (BA) 45/47)**: syntactic processing, working memory.

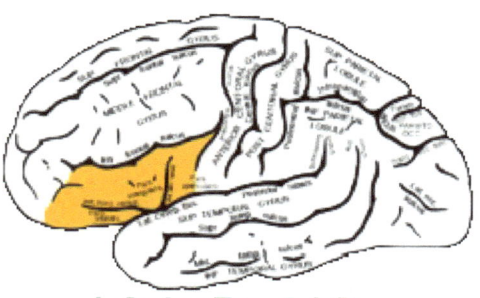
Inferior Frontal Gyrus

- **Inferior frontal gyrus (IFG, BA 44)**: syntactic processing, working memory.

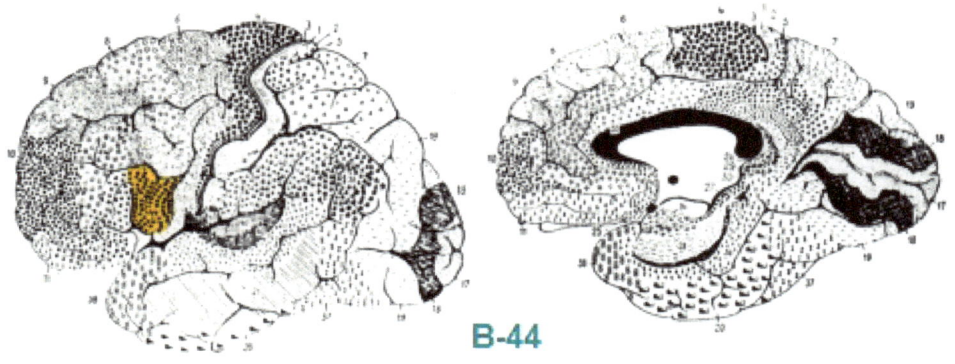
B-44

- **Middle Temporal Gyrus (MTG):** lexical semantic processing.

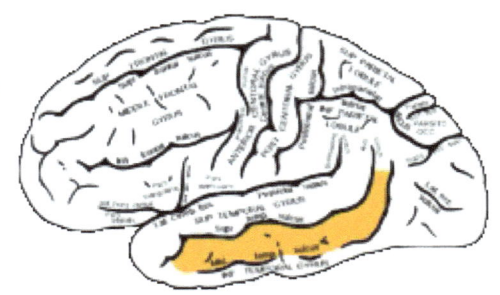

Middle Temporal Gyrus

The left hemisphere is usually dominant in right-handed people, although bilateral activations are not uncommon in the area of syntactic processing. It is now accepted that the right hemisphere plays an important role in the processing of suprasegmental acoustic features, like prosody.

The differentiation of speech production into only two large sections of the brain (Broca's and Wernicke's areas), accepted long before the advent of medical imaging techniques, is now considered outdated.

However, Broca's Area is today still considered an important motor speech center, playing a central role in processing syntax, grammar, and sentence structure. It is named for Pierre Paul Broca (1824-80), a

French anatomist and surgeon. The motor nerves leading to the neck and face, control movements of the tongue, lips, and jaws.

The language recognition center is situated in the right hemisphere. Thus a person who loses the capacity for speech still may be able to understand what is spoken to him or her and vice versa. Damage to Wernicke's area, which is located in the lower part of the temporal lobe, leads mainly to disruptions in speech reception. This area is named for German physician Carl Wernicke (1848-1905), who discovered it in 1874 in the course of his research into aphasia.

Knowing that Wernicke's area is in the front of the auditory cortex could also provide clinical insights into patients suffering from brain damage, such as stroke, or in speech comprehension disorders.

PROSODY

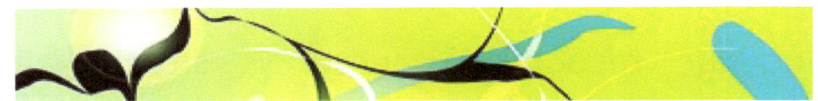

Prosody (from Greek *prosōidía*, pronunciation of syllable) is the *rhythm*, *stress*, and *intonation* of speech. Prosody may reflect various features of speech or the utterance: the emotional state of the speaker; the form of the utterance (statement, question, or command), the presence of irony or sarcasm, emphasis, contrast, and focus, or other elements of language that may not be encoded by grammar or choice of vocabulary.

Producing these nonverbal elements requires intact motor areas of the face, mouth, tongue, and throat. This area is associated with Brodmann areas 44 and 45 of the left frontal lobe. Damage to areas 44/45 produces motor *aprosodia*, with the nonverbal elements of speech being disturbed (facial expression, tone, rhythm of voice).

Understanding these nonverbal elements requires an intact and properly functioning right-hemisphere perisylvian area, particularly Brodmann area 22.

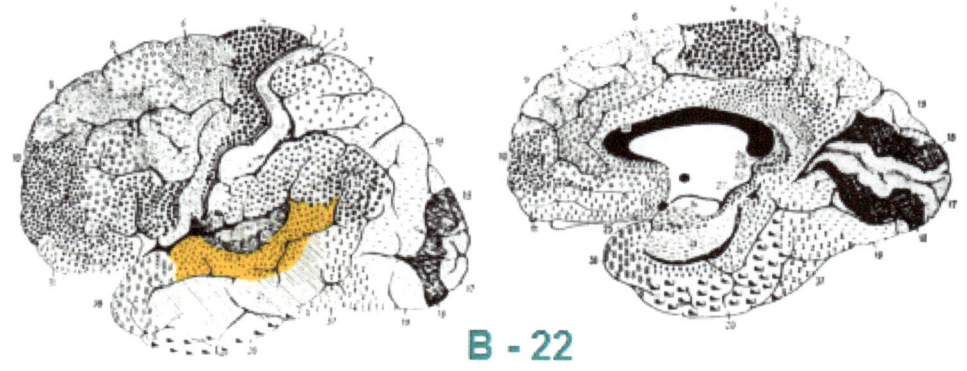

B - 22

Damage to the right inferior frontal gyrus causes a diminished ability to convey emotion or emphasis by voice or gesture, and damage to right superior temporal gyrus causes problems comprehending emotion or emphasis in the voice or gestures of others. The right Brodmann area 22 aids in the interpretation of prosody, and damage causes sensory aprosodia, with the patient unable to comprehend changes in voice and body language.

In terms of acoustics, the prosodics of oral languages involve variation in *syllable length*, *loudness* and *pitch*. In sign languages, prosody involves the *rhythm*, *length*, and *tension of gestures*, along with *mouthing* and *facial expressions*.[19]

Prosody is typically absent in writing, which can occasionally result in reader misunderstanding. Orthographic conventions to mark or substitute for prosody include punctuation (commas, exclamation marks, question marks, scare quotes, and ellipses), and typographic styling for emphasis (italic, bold, and underlined text).

The details of a language's prosody depend upon its phonology. In a language with phonemic vowel length, this must be marked separately from prosodic syllable length. Although tone languages such as Mandarin have prosodic pitch variations in the course of a sentence, such variations are long and smooth contours, on which the short and sharp lexical tones are superimposed. If pitch can be compared to ocean waves, the swells are the prosody, and the wind-blown ripples in their surface are the lexical tones, as with stress in English.

Emotional prosody is the expression of feelings using prosodic elements of speech. It was considered by Charles Darwin in *"The Descent of Man"* to predate the evolution of human language: *"Even monkeys express strong feelings in different tones – anger and impatience by low, – fear and pain by high notes."* [20]

Native speakers listening to actors reading emotionally neutral text while projecting emotions correctly recognize happiness 62% of the time, anger 95%, surprise 91%, sadness 81%, and neutral tone 76%. When a database of this speech is processed by computer, segmental features allow better than 90% recognition of happiness and anger, while suprasegmental prosodic features allow only 44%–49% recognition. The reverse is true for surprise, which is recognized only 69% of the time by segmental features and 96% of the time by suprasegmental prosody.[21]

In typical conversation (no actor voice involved), the recognition of emotion may be quite low, of the order of 50%, hampering the complex interrelationship function of speech advocated by some authors. That said, even if emotional expression through prosody cannot always be consciously recognized, tone of voice may continue to have subconscious effects in conversation. This sort of expression stems from not linguistic or semantic effects, and can thus be isolated from traditional linguistic content.

Aptitude of the average person to decode conversational implicative of emotional prosody has been found to be slightly less accurate than traditional facial expression discrimination ability; however, specific ability to decode varies by emotion. These emotional have been determined to be ubiquitous across cultures, as they are utilized and understood across cultures. Various emotions, and their general experimental identification rates, are as follows:

- **Anger and sadness:** High rate of accurate identification
- **Fear and happiness:** Medium rate of accurate identification
- **Disgust:** Poor rate of accurate identification.

The prosody of an utterance is used by listeners to guide decisions about the emotional affect of the situation. Whether a person decodes the prosody as positive, negative, or neutral plays a factor in the way a person decodes a facial expression accompanying an utterance. As the facial expression becomes closer to neutral, the prosodic interpretation influences the interpretation of the facial expression.

A study revealed that 600 ms of prosodic information is necessary for listeners to be able to identify the affective tone of the utterance. At lengths below this, there is not enough information for listeners to process the emotional context of the utterance.[19]

An *aprosodia* is an acquired or developmental impairment in comprehending or generating the emotion conveyed in speech. Often observed in persons with Asperger syndrome, it is accompanied by the inability to properly utilize variations in speech, accurately modulate pitch, loudness, intonation, and rhythm of word formation.

APHASIA

The loss of the power of speech or the loss of ability to understand verbal or written speech is called *aphasia*. It is a disturbance of language affecting *production*, *comprehension*, *reading or writing*, due to brain injury – most commonly from stroke or trauma. The type of aphasia depends on the brain area affected. A topological model classifies *aphasia* by major characteristics, and links these to areas of the brain in which the damage has been caused. The initial two categories are named after Paul Broca and Carl Wernicke. Other researchers have added a model, named the "Boston-Neoclassical Model".[22]

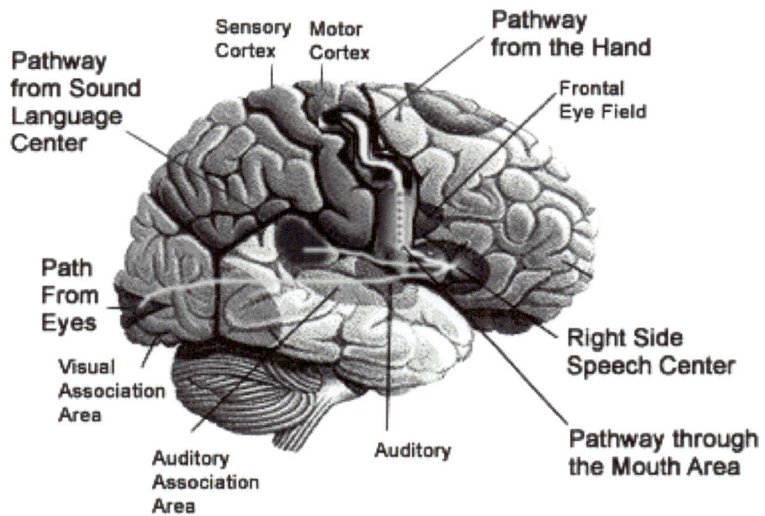

- Broca's aphasia (also called expressive aphasia) is in effect when

Broca's area of the motor speech in the frontal lobe, as well as the medial insular cortex are damaged. The patient has difficulties moving the tongue or facial muscles to produce the sounds of speech. The individual can still read and understand spoken language but has difficulty in speaking and writing. Individuals with expressive aphasia often have right-sided weakness or paralysis of the arm and leg, because of the damage of the frontal lobe.

- In contrast to expressive aphasia, during Wernicke's aphasia (when Wernicke's area is damaged) the individual may speak in long sentences that have no meaning, add unnecessary words, and even create new words. Wernick's aphasia is therefore also called a *fluent aphasia* or *receptive aphasia* (also known as *sensory aphasia*). Patients suffering from receptive aphasia, produce speech without any grammatical problem. However, because the Wernicke's area - that is responsible for language comprehension is damaged, *receptive aphasia* patients cannot convey the meaning. These individuals usually have no body weakness.

Working from Wernicke's model of aphasia, Ludwig Lichtheim

proposed five other types of aphasia, but these were not tested against real patients until modern imaging made more in-depth studies available. The other five types of aphasia in the localization model are:

- *Auditory verbal agnosia* (also known as *Pure Word Deafness*)
- *Conduction aphasia*
- *Apraxia of speech* (now considered a separate disorder in itself)
- *Transcortical motor aphasia* (also known as *Adynamic aphasia* or *Extrasylvian motor aphasia*), and
- *Transcortical sensory aphasia.*

Anomic aphasia, also known as anomia or *dysnomia,* is another type of aphasia proposed under what is commonly known as the *Boston-Neoclassical model.*

Global aphasia results from damage to extensive portions of the perisylvian region of the brain. An individual with global aphasia will have difficulty understanding both spoken and written language and will also have difficulty speaking. This is a severe type of aphasia which makes communication a challenge.

Isolation aphasia, also known as *mixed transcortical aphasia,* is a type of disturbance that causes the inability to comprehend what is being said or the difficulty in creating speech with meaning, without affecting the ability to recite what has been said and to acquire newly presented words. This type of aphasia is caused by brain damage that isolates the parts of the brain from other parts that are in charge of speech. *Isolation aphasia* patients can not produce meaningful speech of their own.

There are also other speech disorders, such as *dysarthria, dysphonia,* not necessarily associated with the damage to the speech centers.

Dysarthria is a defect in the articulation and rhythm of speech because of weakness in the muscles that form words. Amyotrophic lateral sclerosis (Lou Gehrig's disease) and myasthenia gravis are two diseases with which such muscle weakness can be associated.

Dysphonia is a hoarseness of the voice that can be caused by a brain tumor or any number of non-neurologic factors. [23]

POLYGLOTISM AND SAVANT SYNDROME

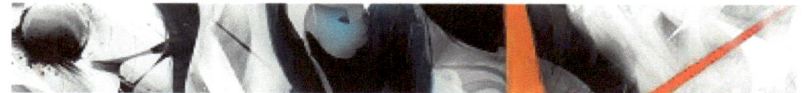

Polyglotism is a term for a multilingual person who can master more than three languages.

Numerous theories exist as explanations for polyglotism, among them a theory suggesting that a spike in a baby's testosterone levels while in the uterus can increase brain asymmetry, while others have suggested that hard work and the right type of motivation—which any adult can apply—are the key factors of polyglotism.[24]

Neuroscientist Katrin Amunts studied the brain of German polyglot Emil Krebs and determined that the area of Krebs' brain that was responsible for the motor language—the Broca's area—was organized differently in comparison to the brains of monolinguals.

Due to the advent of computers, linguists obtained a better understanding of what it can mean to *"know a language fluently"*. It is estimated that the most frequently used 2000 words—in all or most of their multiple senses—cover approximately 75% to 80% of a general text in English and other European languages; such a limited vocabulary also allows one to express more complicated concepts, whereby they are described by means of circumlocutions (as a rule, 30,000 to 50,000 words in modern English learner's dictionaries are defined with merely 2000 to 3000 defining vocabulary words).

On the other hand, a native speaker with an American college education may possess a 25,000- to 30,000-word passive vocabulary—of which various parts can be activated—that increases to possibly 50,000 words, or more, by the age of fifty to sixty years. It is therefore difficult to objectively judge many claims of polyglotism, as what is ostensibly "fluent speech" can be achieved with the assertive use of a very limited general-purpose or specialized vocabulary.

In order to achieve electro-physiological measures of language processing in bilinguals, *event-related brain potentials* (ERPs) were recorded from right-handed polyglots and monolinguals during a task involving silent reading. The stimuli were terminal words that would correctly complete a short, meaningful, previously shown sentence, or else were semantically or syntactically incorrect. The task consisted in deciding whether the sentences were well formed or not, giving the response by pressing a button.

For the bilinguals, the ERP results revealed a strong, left-sided activation, reflected by the N1 component, of the occipital-temporal regions dedicated to orthographic processing, with a latency of about 150 msec for Slovenian words, but bilateral activation of the same areas for Italian words, which was also displayed by topographical mapping.

In monolinguals, semantic error produced a long-lasting negative response (N2 and N4) that was greater over the right hemisphere, whereas syntactic error activated mostly the left hemisphere. Conversely, in the bilinguals, semantic incongruence resulted in greater response over the left hemisphere than over the right. In this group, the P615 syntactical error responses were of equal amplitude on both hemispheres for Italian words and greater on the right side for Slovenian words.

Findings of this study support the view that there are interand intrahemispheric brain activation asymmetries when monolingual and bilingual speakers comprehend written language. The fact that the bilingual speakers are highly fluent and had acquired both languages in early infancy, suggests that the brain activation patterns do not depend on the age of acquisition or the fluency level, as in the case of late, not-so-proficient L2 language learners, but on the functional organization of the bilinguals' brain due to polyglotism and based on brain plasticity.[25]

Savants are individuals with serious mental illnesses who demonstrate profound and prodigious capacities or abilities far in excess of what would be considered normal, including the capacity for languages.

While polyglot savants such as Emil Krebs may have anatomical or biological differences that allow them to organize language in a different and more efficient manner, it has also been suggested that the entire language acquisition process for polyglot savants is different than the process most humans undergo.

It has been proposed that these individuals with unparalleled linguistic abilities undergo the same first language acquisition process over and over again with each new language. Because they are able to consciously or unconsciously learn the pragmatics, grammar, syntax of a language as if they were learning a language for the first time, they are able to acquire it as proficiently as a native speaker.[26]

People with savant syndrome may also have

neurodevelopmental disorders, notably autism spectrum disorders or brain injuries. The most dramatic examples are seen in individuals who score very low on IQ tests, while demonstrating exceptional skills or brilliance in specific areas, such as rapid calculation, art, memory, or musical ability.

There are two forms of the savant syndrome: the congenital and acquired forms. Among the many examples of the congenital form are the calendar calculators, who can quickly provide the day of the week for any date in the past. Other examples are the musical savants with perfect pitch and the hyperlexics, who can read a page in 8 seconds and recall the text later at a 99% level. Other types of talents and artistic skills can be found, involving 3-D drawing, map memory, poetry, painting, sculpturing, including one savant who could recite without error the value of Pi to 22,514 places.

The acquired form refers to the development of outstanding skills after some brain injury or disease, usually involving the left frontal-temporal area. This type of injury seems to inhibit the *'tyranny of the left hemisphere,'* allowing the right hemisphere to develop the savant skills. One other way to inhibit the left frontal-temporal area is to use transcranial magnetic stimulation in normal subjects and nearly one-half of these subjects can then perform new skills during the stimulation that they could not perform before. This type of finding indicates the potentiality in all of us for the development of savant skills under special circumstances. Explanations of the congenital savant syndrome include *enhanced local connectivity* as a compensation for under-connectivity of long-range fibers, but also *weak central coherence*, replaced by *great attention to details*, *enhanced perceptual functioning* and *obsessive pre-occupation with specific interests.*[27]

Most humans allow the grammar of previously learned languages affect and influence their ability to learn a second, third, etc. language. This is an issue that these polyglot savants do not struggle with. This ability may be tied directly to how these individuals organize Broca's area of the brain however; their learning abilities for languages are unparalleled and still not 100% understood to this day.

A study utilized a high-resolution MRI, J-resolved MR spectroscopy, and diffusion tensor imaging data for a single scanning session of a 63-year-old male autistic savant with prodigious artistic skills. Regional and compartmental brain volumes, N-acetyl aspartate, choline, creatine, glutamate and γ-aminobutyric acid concentrations, fractional anisotropy values, and white matter bundle volumes as well as axial, radial, and mean diffusivities were calculated. No gross anatomical differences were observed. By morphological assessment, cerebral volume (1362 mL) was larger than normative literature values for adult males. The corpus callosum was intact and did not exhibit abnormal structural features. The right cerebral hemisphere was 1.9% larger than the left hemisphere; the right amygdala and right caudate nuclei were 24% and 9.9% larger, respectively, compared with the left side. In contrast, the putamen was 8.3% larger on the left side. Fiber tract bundle volumes were larger on the right side for the amygdala, hippocampus, frontal lobe, and occipital lobe. Both the left and the right hippocampi had substantially increased axial and mean diffusivities as compared with those of a comparison sample of nonsavant adult males. The corpus callosum and left amygdala also exhibited high axial, radial, and mean diffusivities. MR spectroscopy revealed markedly decreased γ-aminobutyric acid and glutamate in the parietal lobe.[28]

There is still much research that needs to be done regarding the mechanisms through which polyglot savants acquire language. Although it is apparent that polyglot savants have amazing linguistic abilities, quite often their general intellectual ability is impaired. Poor hand-eye coordination, weak problem solving abilities, and social and conversational problems, make every day tasks very difficult for the polyglots. [29]

Tom Wiggins (blind pianist), Alonzo Clemons (composer), Tony DeBlois (sculptor), Jason Hughes (blind musician), Leslie Lemke (sociologist), Jonathan Lerman (blind musician), James Henry Pullen (author), Matt Savage (carpenter), Henriett Seth (jazz prodigy), Richard Wawro (architect), Jason Padgett (blind pianist), and many others are known as the savant geniuses.

PHYSIOLOGY OF THE S.M.A.R.T. SPEECH

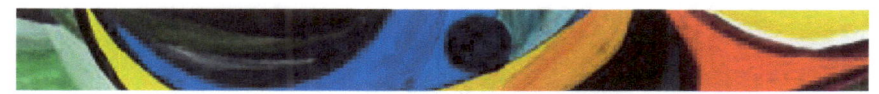

There are so many terms and syndromes linked to the speech producing process that one may wonder, whether the S.M.A.R.T speech is a physiological or 'pathological' phenomenon?

Speech production is a complex process, involving a networked system of brain areas that each contribute in unique ways. The ability to produce accurate speech sounds in rapid succession is something we humans take for granted.

In the extremely involving process of speech production, thoughts must be translated into linguistic representations (itself not a trivial feat), which are then sent to speech mechanisms that can coordinate, initiate, modify and execute the articulation of an utterance. Numerous brain areas are recruited in speech production and they are only a few centimeters apart to each other. They hang in a precarious balance that is easily affected by neurological disease and dysfunction.

Given the number of sophisticated movements that are

required for speech production, it is no wonder that the mouth area is so largely represented in the homunculus of primary motor cortex. Patients with deficits in this ability to programme speech movements are said to have a *'apraxia of speech'* disorder.

While there is an ample evidence about the anatomy and topology of the speech producing centers in the brain, yet there are no descriptions of physiology of the state -of-art speech production.

Specific speech: Here, the term "specific" is different from the known Specific Speech and Language Impairment (SSLI) disability which is usually observed in early childhood. Numbers of brain centers are involved to produce a specified speech: among them the *Wernicke's area* and of course, the *frontal lobe* - responsible for the reasoning, planning, creativity, judgment, problem solving, and planning.

Meaningful speech: The *temporal lobes* are responsible for hearing, memory, meaning, and language. They are concerned with interpreting and processing auditory stimuli. They also play a role in emotion and learning.

"If you want me to speak for two minutes, it will take me three weeks of

preparation. If you want me to speak for thirty minutes, it will take me a week to prepare. If you want me to speak for an hour, I am ready now, " Winston Churchill.

Articulate speech: It is when the speaker utters clearly in distinct syllables, uses language easily and fluently; has facility with words, expressed, formulated, or presented with clarity and effectiveness. Thus, the process of producing an articulate speech requires verbal intelligence, adequate vocabulary, knowledge and experience. It is not necessarily related with creativity or planning. The process toward literacy mimics the process of oral language development.

The brain regions involved in coordinating an articulate speech, remain largely unknown. A study located brain lesions of 25 stroke patients with a disorder in the motor planning of articulatory movements, and compared those with lesions of 19 patients without such deficits. A robust double dissociation was found between these two groups. All patients with articulatory planning deficits had lesions that included a discrete region of the left precentral gyms of the *insula*, the cortical area beneath the frontal and temporal lobes. This area was completely spared in all patients without these articulation deficits. Thus this area seems to be specialized for the motor planning of speech.[30-32]

Relevant speech: Language is systematic, predictable and redundant. It allows us to categorize, organize and retrieve information. Language involves two processes: the message (vocabulary and comprehension), and the way the message is delivered (phonemic awareness, phonics and fluency). Written language is the graphic code used to convey the message of the oral language. Listening and reading involve receiving messages. Talking and writing involve giving messages.

Relevance is the comprehension or production of the message intent. It is known that the *occipital lobe* is involved with the brain's ability to recognize objects. Thus, it may be equally responsible for grasping the intent and relevance of the message.

A study mapped the brain systems engaged during propositional speech (PrSp) and two forms of non- propositional speech (NPrSp): counting and reciting overlearned nursery rhymes. Bilateral cerebral and cerebellar regions were involved in the motor act of articulation, irrespective of the type of speech. Three additional, left-lateral regions, adjacent to the *Sylvian sulcus*, were activated in common: the most posterior part of the supratemporal plane, the lateral part of the pars opercularis in the posterior inferior frontal gyrus and the anterior insula. [33]

Therefore, both NPrSp and PrSp are dependent on the same discrete subregions of the anatomically ill-defined areas of Wernicke and Broca. PrSp is also dependent on a predominantly left-lateralized neural system distributed between multi-modal and amodal regions in posterior inferior parietal, anterolateral and medial *temporal* and *medial prefrontal cortex*. The lateral prefrontal and paracingulate cortical activity observed in previous studies of cued word retrieval is not seen with either NPrSp or PrSp, demonstrating that normal and relevant language representations cannot be inferred from explicit metalinguistic tasks.

These findings indicate that normal communicative speech is dependent on a number of left hemisphere regions remote from the classic language areas of Wernicke and Broca. Destruction or disconnection of discrete *left extrasylvian* and *perisylvian cortical regions*, rather than the total extent of damage to *perisylvian cortex*, will account for the qualitative and quantitative differences.

Time-bound speech: A meaningful speech cannot be abstract. Abstract are the timeless concepts, such as happiness, love, crime, freedom, hope, home, or help. In order a speech be smart and convincing, it has to be measurable, and must uncover the concept in relevance with the definite time period. It must present the background and history of the concept and appreciate why that concept is relevant to the audience. time-bounding speech would simplify contents and examples to the point, where we find it easy to apply or connect with the subject from our points of view.

For example: *"I love to be free"* announcement would seem pointless and boring for the audience, for it has two abstract concepts. Simplifying and pushing the concept closer to the recipient, it would sound like this: *"Now that our lives are computerized and we get the necessary information momentarily, we all have more free time to devote on things we enjoy."* The second statement again, is too abstract; however it has some time-bounding element.

Simplifying and time-bound speech requires a lot of brain-work. It involves the two hemispheres, for it includes inference and iteration. In the right-handed individuals the time-bounding speech involves the right hemisphere for the spatial tasks and object recognition. In the same individuals, it also involves the left hemisphere for the semantic functions and projections. Thus, the time-bounding speech is the product of the complex network, comprised of the seven regions: *posterior inferior parietal lobe*, *middle temporal gyrus*, *fusiform and parahippocampal gyri*, *dorsomedial prefrontal cortex*, *inferior frontal gyrus*, *ventromedial prefrontal cortex*, and *posterior cingulate gyrus.* Secondary analyses shows specific subregions of this network associated with knowledge of actions, manipulable artifacts, abstract concepts, and concrete concepts.

The MRI studies reveal that the cortical regions involved in semantic processing can be grouped into the three broad categories: *posterior multimodal* and *heteromodal association cortex*, *heteromodal prefrontal cortex*, and *medial limbic regions.* [34]

CONCLUSIONS

S.M.A.R.T speech is a complex, creative process and a succession involving a networked system of brain areas that each contribute in unique ways. To produce a specific, meaningful, articulate, relevant, and time-bound speech, the individual recruits and utilizes the potential of uncountable cerebral areas from the both hemispheres, insula, stem, and cerebellum. At this stage, with the help of neuroimaging techniques, the following areas are defined to be responsible in producing a S.M.A.R.T. speech:

Specific speech	S	*Frontal lobe, Wernicke's area*
Meaningful speech	M	*Temporal lobes*
Articulate speech	A	*Insula, Broca's area*
Relevant speech	R	*Sylvian sulcus, Perisylvian cortex, Left extrasylvian cortex, Broca's area, Wernicke's area, Temporal cortex, Medial Prefrontal cortex*
Time-bound speech	T	*Dorsomedial prefrontal cortex, Fusiform and Parahippocampal gyri, Heteromodal prefrontal cortex, Inferior frontal gyrus, Medial limbus, Middle temporal gyrus, Posterior cingulate gyrus, Posterior inferior parietal lobe, Posterior multimodal cortex, Ventromedial prefrontal cortex*

Be smart and simple!

INDEX OF TERMS

Term	Abbreviation	Page [s]
Amygdala		39
Anomia		31
Aphasia		23, 29, 30-32
Apraxia		31, 42
Aprosodia		24, 25, 28
Area frontalis agranularis	AFA	20
Blood-oxygen-level-dependent	BOLD	20
Boston-Neoclassical Model	BNM	29, 31
Broca's area	BrA	22, 29, 30, 33, 38, 45, 48
Brodmann areas- 6, 22, 44, 45, 47	BA	20, 21, 24, 25
Central limit theorem	CLT	10
Dorsomedial prefrontal cortex	DPC	48
Dysarthria		32
Dysphonia		32
Enhanced local connectivity	ELC	38
Event-related brain potentials	ERPs	34
Functional magnetic resonance imaging	f-MRI	20, 37, 48
Fusiform gyrus	FG	48

γ-aminobutyric acid	**GAA**	39
Gaussian difficulty	**G-d**	9, 10, 12, 15
Heteromodal prefrontal cortex	**HPC**	48
Inferior frontal gyrus	**IFG**	20, 21, 25, 45, 47
Insula		43, 45, 48
Limbic system		47, 48
MacArthur-Bates communicative development inventory	**MCDI**	6
McMurray model		9, 18
Middle temporal gyrus	**MTG**	22
Multimodal cortex	**MC**	48
N-acetyl aspartate	**NAA**	39
Negative binomial random variable	**NBRV**	15
Non- propositional speech	**NPrSp**	44, 45
Nuclei caudate	**NC**	20, 39
Polyglotism		33, 34, 36
Positron emission tomography	**PET**	20
Posterior cingulate gyrus	**PCG**	47, 48
Prefrontal cortex		45, 47, 48
Perisylvian cortex		45, 48
Prosody		22, 24-28

Propositional speech	**PrSp**	44, 45
Putamen		20, 39
Savant syndrome	**SS**	33, 37, 38, 40
Stochastic simulation method		9, 11, 15, 28, 19
Specific speech & language impairment	**SSLI**	42
Superior temporal gyrus	**STG**	20, 21
Sylvian sulcus		44, 48
Testosterone	**Ts**	33
Vocabulary spurt		3, 5, 6, 8, 9
Ventromedial prefrontal cortex	**VPC**	48
Wernicke's area	**WA**	19, 22, 23, 29, 30, 42, 45, 48

WORKS CITED:

(1) **Hoff E (2005).** *Language experience and language milestones during early childhood.* In K. McCartney & D. Phillips (Eds). Blackwell Handbook of early childhood development: Blackwell Publishing, Blackwell reference online. (Paperback).

(2) **Clark E V, Grossman J B (1998).** *Pragmatics directions and children's word learning.* Journal of Child Language 25 (1): 1–18

(3) **Keren-Portnoy T, Majorano M, Vihman M M. (2009).** *From phonetics to phonology: The emergence of first words in Italian.* Journal of Child Language 36 (2): 235–267

(4) **Ganger J, Brent MR (2004).** *Reexamining the vocabulary spurt.* Developmental Psychology 40 (4): 621–632

(5) **Hulit LM, Howard MR (2002).** *Born to talk.* Toronto: Allyn and Bacon (Hardcover).

(6) **Dale P, Fenson L. (1996).** *Lexical development norms for young children.* Behavior Research Methods, Instruments,& Computers, 28, 125-127.

(7) **Lorraine S (2008).** *Vocabulary development: Super duper handouts number 149.* Greenville, SC: Super Duper Publications (Hardcover)

(8) **Anglin JM, Miller GA (2000).** *Vocabulary development: A morphological analysis.* Wiley-Blackwell (Paperback)

(9) **Gopnik A, Meltzoff A N. (1987).** *The development of categorization in the second year and its relation to other cognitive and linguistic developments.* Child Development, 58, 1523-1531

(10) **Reznick JS, Goldfield B.A. (1992).** *Rapid change in lexical development in comprehension and production.* Developmental Psychology,28, 406413.

(11) **Gleitman LR, Gleitman H. (1992).** *A picture is worth a thousand words, but thats the problem: the role of syntax in vocabulary acquisition.* Current Directions in Psychological Science, 1, 31-5.

(12) **Markman EM, Wasow JL, Hanson MB (2003).** *Use of the mutual exclusivity assumption by young word learners.* Cognitive Psychology, 47, 241-275.

(13) **Plunkett K (1993).** *Lexical segmentation and vocabulary growth in early language acquisition.* Journal of Child Language, 20, 4360.

(14) **van Geert P. (1991).** *A dynamic systems model of cognitive and language growth.* Psychological Review, 98, 353.

(15) **McMurray B, Mitchell CC (2007).** *A stochastic model for the vocabulary explosion.* Department Of Mathematics and Department of Psychology; University of Iowa

(16) **Friederici AD (2002).** *Towards a neural basis of auditory sentence processing.* Trends in Cognitive Sciences; 6:78

(17) **Kandel ER, Schwartz JH, Jessel TM (2000).** *Principles of neuroscience.* Fourth Edition, New York: McGraw-Hill: 1169–1187

(18) **Donald Loritz (1999).** *How the Brain evolved Language.* Oxford University Press (Hardcover)

(19) **Pell MD (2005).** *Prosody–face interactions in emotional processing as revealed by the facial affect decision task.* Journal of Nonverbal Behavior; 29 (4): 193–215

(20) **Darwin C (1871).** *Descent of man.* Wallace (Hardcover)

(21) **Miller LA, Collins RL, Kent TA (2008).** *Language and the modulation of impulsive aggression.* The Journal of neuropsychiatry and clinical neurosciences; 20 (3): 261–73

(22) **Kolb B, Ian Q. (2003).** *Fundamentals of human neuropsychology.* (NY, Paperback)

(23) **Carlson N (2007).** *Psychology the Science of Behaviour.* Toronto: Pearson. (Paperback)

(24) **Leland J (2012).** *Adventures of a teenage polyglot.* The New York Times, March 9

(25) **Proverbio AM, Cok B, Zani A (2002).** *Electrophysiological measures of language processing in bilinguals.* Journal of Cognitive Neurscience; 1;14(7):994-1017

(26) **Bolte S (2004).** *Comparing the intelligence profiles of savant and nonsavant individuals with autistic disorder.* Intelligence; 32 (2): 121

(27) **Hughes JR (2012).** *The savant syndrome and its possible relationship to epilepsy.* Advances of Experimental Medicine and Biology; 724:332-43

(28) **Corrigan NM, Richards TL, Treffert DA, Dager SR (2012).** *Toward a better understanding of the savant brain.* Comprehensive Psychiatry; 53(6):706-17

(29) **Yamaguchi M (2011).** *Call for more rigorous research on savant syndrome.* Archives of Medical Science;7(6):1085-6

(30) **Blumstein S (1991).** *Acquired aphasia,* 2nd ed. Academic, San Diego

(31) **Johns DF, Darley FL (1970).** *Speech.* Hearing Research; 13, 556–583

(32) **Shankweiler D, Harris KS (1966).** *Cortex;* 2, 277–292

(33) **Black SC, Scott SK, Murphy K, et al (2002).** *Speech production: Wernicke, Broca and beyond.* Brain: A journal of Neurology; 125 (8): 1829-1838

(34) **Binder JR, Desai RH, Graves WW, Conant LL (2009).** *Where is the semantic system? A critical review and meta-analysis of 120 functional neuroimaging studies.* Cerebral cortex; 19 (12): 2767-2796

www.ingramcontent.com/pod-product-compliance
Lightning Source LLC
Chambersburg PA
CBHW050812180526
45159CB00004B/1639